Six Pack Abs Diet and Exercise Plan

5 Exercises and 5 Meals to Bust Belly Fat and Get That Six Pack You've Always Wanted

Kelsey James

Green Ribbon Engagements, LLC. ©2015

Disclaimer

TABLE OF CONTENTS

Introduction

Do you struggle with excess belly fat?

Have you tried everything and still can't shed those last few pounds?

Are you ready to finally get that six-pack you have always dreamed of?

If you have always fantasized about having a stomach that celebrity trainers would be jealous of while never having to worry about fitting into your favorite jeans then this book can help you achieve all of your goals when it comes to ridding your belly of extra and annoying fat.

5 Exercises and 5 Meals to Bust Belly Fat reveals tried and true techniques that will allow you to easily shed those last few pounds above your waist while still enjoying delicious food, including comfort foods like pasta and pizza. You will unlock the secrets to shedding belly fat and sculpting your stomach muscles into an ideal six pack that everyone at the beach will staring at. You will learn what belly fat really is and what causes it to accumulate. You will also discover some of the many reasons that may be preventing you from losing the extra weight in your midsection. You will learn step-by-step exercises that will blast away pounds, burn calories and leave you with defined muscles.

These exercises will also make you aware of how your current workout routine may be doing nothing to help you achieve your goals. You will learn recipes with ingredients that have natural fat blasting properties and you may even be surprised at how delicious eating right can be.

The best part about this book is that these solutions are not temporary or just a quick fix. You will learn how to keep belly fat at bay for the rest of your life without spending every hour at the gym and counting every calorie.

This is because what you about to learn are not just metaphorical Band-Aids for your problem with belly fat. They are the solution that you have been searching for.

So if you are ready, stop doing crunches, put down the celery stick and learn how to once and for all get rid of your love handles and be confident when walking down the beach, showing off your new six-pack of abs.

Chapter 1

The Stomach Struggle is Real

What exactly is belly fat?

Many people struggle with shedding unwanted pounds, especially when it comes to the ones that are found in the stomach region. While the first few pounds may come off easily for some, there always seems to be an impossible hurdle to jump when trying to lose the final pounds. This extra and stubborn weight is usually located around the midsection and not only leads to a dip in self esteem but is also incredibly dangerous to one's health.

There are three different types of fat that are present and necessary in the human body. Fats not only provide the body with a concentrated form of energy but they are necessary for the body to transport and absorb certain vitamins. Some fats cannot be produced within the body and therefore need to be consumed in healthy amounts.

Triglycerides are the fat found in the bloodstream. When a person eats, the calories that the body does not use immediately as energy are converted into triglycerides. They are then stored as a type of energy reserve that can be used in between meals and snacks. They are the most common type of body fat, making up ninety-five percent of all the fat in the body.

Subcutaneous fat is the immediate layer of fat found below the outer layer of skin. This is the body's form of padding and also acts as insulation to keep the body warm. It also serves as an energy reserve if other forms of energy are unavailable for the body to use.

Finally, there is visceral fat, commonly referred to as belly fat. This type of fat is found deep in the abdominal cavity, beneath all of the stomach muscles. It is a very dangerous type of fat and can also be the hardest to get rid of. While it may cause an individual to feel unattractive, it has much more serious consequences. Visceral fat has been linked to being a contributing factor in the development of type 2 diabetes, heart disease, breast cancer, colorectal cancer and Alzheimer's disease.

Even if a person is thin, they can still have a surplus of visceral fat in their abdominal cavity. Since it is located and stored under the muscles, it can be hard to determine if the amount is healthy or dangerous. The most reliable and accurate measurement of this fat is to view it on an MRI scan, but this is certainly not the most affordable or convenient test. A general test administered by the medical field is a waistline measurement.

Men should have a waist measurement of no more than 40 inches, while women should have a measurement of 35 inches or less. If a person's waist measurement is more than the number recommended for their sex, there is a large chance that the visceral fat content in their body is dangerously high and they should immediately begin a regimen to decrease the amount.

When Dieting Isn't Working

Most people try to tackle losing belly weight by going on a strict diet and completing countless sit-ups. The problem with this method though is that this specific type of fat needs to be tackled in a more direct fashion. The same exercise routine that allowed them to lose other weight will simply not have the same effect on belly fat. Their workout will need to increase in intensity and target all of their core muscles simultaneously. Since the fat is underneath the muscles in the stomach, crunches are not an effective exercise and will never produce the results that a person is after.

Cutting calories is usually great for weight loss. However, if the type of calories that are still being consumed are feeding the fat then there will be no weight loss and the individual may actually gain pounds. One should avoid giving themselves a set number of calories that they are allowed to consume each day. Instead, they focus on eating healthier foods that will provide their body with the nutrients and healthy fats that it needs to function properly.

Other Factors Adding Belly Fat

There may be other factors that are playing a role in a person's weight struggle that will take more patience and planning to overcome. Age can play a large role in the stomach's appearance. As the body ages, it is natural that its metabolism slows down and weight becomes easier to put on. This can be incredibly common in women going through menopause. The shift in hormones causes any extra weight to collect in the midsection. While this is frustrating, it is fixable.

If an individual is stressed (and with today's hectic lifestyles mostly everyone is) the hormone called cortisol will be present in higher amounts in the bloodstream. This is necessary to help the body combat stress but it also causes the body to store fat and protect it. It will also allow the fat cells to grow bigger. A lack of sleep can also cause belly weight gain. Studies show that adults getting less than six hours of sleep will generally weigh more than adults getting seven to eight hours of rest a night.

Is society doomed to suffer with belly fat forever then?

Absolutely not.

With a workout routine that includes effective and intense exercises combined with a menu of healthy meals, the weight will start to come off and the formation of six pack abs will begin.

Chapter 2

What is a Six Pack?

The road to a six-pack is long and hard. Eating right and exercising take commitment. Achieving desired results is more than just physical work. There has to be some education as well. Their needs to be a firm understanding of what a set of six pack abs *actually* is. The anatomy of the human abdomen is complex and contains many more muscles than people realize, which contributes to the difficulty of getting that dream six pack. Most people only work out a few of the muscles, and even complete their exercises incorrectly or inefficiently.

Sometimes, it's noticeable that people's abs look different. Although both movie stars have great midsections, Ryan Reynolds and Hugh Jackman's abs look starkly different. Some people have a six-pack, while some obtain that shredded eight pack look! This doesn't mean that one did fewer workouts while the other put in extra hours at the gym. The difference in appearance is more an example of their individual anatomy and body type than work ethic.

The six pack look is caused when a connective tissue, known as the fascia, is toned through exercises so that it crosses the abdominal muscles tightly, creating the ripple affect that is so coveted. No matter how many or few workouts someone does, they can never change the number of fascia bands that are present in your abdomen.

The anatomy of the midsection is made up of six main muscle groups. Some provide visually appealing results when they are worked out while others provide extra strength and a slimmer waistline.

Abdominal Muscles

Rectus Abdominis

This is the main muscle that will provide someone with a six pack. Starting at the bottom of the sternum, it runs along the whole length of the stomach and inserts into the pelvis. This is the muscle that is primarily used when lifting the knees up and down. Someone may hear abs described as upper or lower, but they are all part of the same muscle, the rectus abdominis.

External Obliques

These muscles run along the sides of the body diagonally. These are the difficult to tone muscles that will really keep the stomach looking trim when properly exercised. Every time someone twists or turns their body they are engaging their external obliques.

Serratus

These muscles run along the top portion of the rib cage. These muscles help to swing the arms and lift heavy objects above the head. If properly toned, they will help frame a tight six pack. Due to their location they can be difficult to target during traditional ab exercises.

Transverse Abdominis

This muscle is hidden underneath the rectus abdominus. It is not a muscle that will provide definition on the outside of the body; however, when this muscle is safely tightened, it can instantly provide the individual with a slimmer waistline. Think of it as nature's girdle.

Internal Obliques

As the name suggests, the internal obliques can be found underneath the external obliques. They are equally important, running in the opposite direction as the external and allowing the body a full range of motion when twisting or turning.

Intercostals

These muscles are located beneath and even in between the rib bones. They aid in breathing by moving the chest wall to allow inspiration and expiration. While breathing is always important during exercise, engaging in a controlled and properly timed breathing pattern when working the abs will also work the intercostals.

When putting together a personal ab workout routine, one will want to make sure that they are targeting all of these muscles. Focusing on each one individually though can be time consuming and exhausting and may cause one to slack on their routine. Therefore, the best bet to achieving a six-pack and sticking to a routine is to find exercises that target multiple areas with enough intensity to give them a workout. All of these muscles are used during daily actions, such as walking, twisting and even breathing. Therefore, one may need to rethink their workout's intensity levels to make sure that they are challenging each muscle group.

Chapter 3

Mental Strength

Emotional Eating

One of the most difficult parts of dieting is being able to keep motivation. Sometimes the brain is the body's worst enemy. Any type of emotion may lead someone to over indulge in foods that can lead to weight gain, especially in the midsection. This emotional and mindless eating plagues many people and is more common than one may think.

The body releases many hormones when it is stressed. The increase in these hormones pushes the body to crave certain types of foods, such as sugar and carbohydrates. When the craving is satisfied, it starts a habit that can be difficult to break. The food is viewed by the body as a distraction to the unpleasant feelings it may be experiencing, like sadness, anger or anxiety. This type of mindless eating can lead to chronic conditions.

Most people may not realize that they are an emotional eater. Some warning signs include experiencing guilt after eating, eating when bored and having strong cravings during emotional times. In order to overcome this vicious cycle, the behavior must first be recognized and then handled appropriately.

Remove any distractions while eating. Avoid watching television or looking at a cell phone. A meal should be an enjoyable experience and by focusing on the taste of the food and appreciating the moment, mindless eating can be avoided.

Pay attention to serving sizes and portion control. Instead of grabbing a box of crackers and eating directly out of it, remove the recommended serving size and evaluate hunger after finishing. This will prevent the consumption of unneeded calories.

Although this may sound obvious, avoid eating just because other people are. This is a common habit at parties or other events where food is present. Only eat if the body is hungry and then choose healthy options.

Mind Power

Mental strength is an important part of weight loss. Emotional or unhealthy eating is a habit that needs to be broken. The behavior of incorrect eating will eventually occur unconsciously and cannot be broken without strong mental influence. The brain will need just as much training as the rest of the body when tackling weight loss.

It will be easier to keep the mind from allowing someone to sidetrack from their diet if they make a list of all the reasons that they want to lose weight. This list should then be kept somewhere where they will see it everyday. This constant exposure to their desires will remind their brain of why they are doing this in the first place. This will retrain the brain in how it views comfort foods and the hard work of exercise.

Set small goals that will provide feelings of accomplishment. These small steps will help to keep motivation levels up and keep the progress on track. Remain positive and avoid negative thoughts. Inner thoughts should not be a discouraging factor when dieting and exercising.

Muscles will get tired and cravings will hit. Success is dependent on the mental reactions to these issues. Focus on the end goal and push any negativity out. This is an important key that most people ignore when starting a new exercise and diet routine.

Chapter 4

Tips for Success

Diets can be difficult and trying. Here are some guidelines and helpful tips that can make the process easier.

<u>Foods to Enjoy</u>

There are some foods that will fuel the body and even help burn fat while some foods should be completely avoided while focusing on eliminating belly fat.

Oatmeal

> This is a fiber rich breakfast food that will keep the stomach full until lunch, helping one to avoid unhealthy snacks. Try adding some fiber packed berries for a little extra flavor.

Protein Powder

Smoothies are a great way to get a healthy meal in when there is little time to prepare a meal. Keep some protein powder around to add to the blender. It contains amino acids that will help build up muscles and also burn fat.

Olive Oil

This is a healthy oil that is better for cooking or as a base for salad dressing. Coconut oil is another great alternative to use during meal preparation.

Lean Meats and Fish

The body actually burns calories while it digests food and will be able to burn more if an individual consumes leaner meats and fish instead of heavy carbohydrates or unhealthy fats.

Whole Grains

It is common knowledge that carbohydrates can corrupt a diet but there are healthier versions that can be consumed to keep cravings at bay. Whole grain breads are full of fiber and nutrients.

Green Vegetables

Salads and other green vegetables are a great way to stay full during the day without consuming excess calories. Always have a salad before dinner to avoid overindulging.

Foods to Avoid

While it is expected to slip a little on a diet during special occasions or as a treat, precautions should be taken to avoid these fat adding foods.

Fructose

Avoid foods that are heavy in fructose, such as apples or honey. These foods will cause the stomach to bloat.

Carbonated Beverages

Not only will carbonation leave someone feeling bloated and gassy, diet soft drinks are directly linked to weight-gain and belly fat.

Refined Carbohydrates

Unlike the healthier whole grain carbohydrates, foods like white bread, crackers and bagels can cause blood sugar to spike. This will lead to a larger waste line.

Alcohol

It is acceptable to still indulge in a drink with dinner, but stick with wine and enjoy in extreme moderation. Beer and spirits are not only high in calories but alcohol can increase one's appetite which may cause them to make unhealthy choices.

Daily Tips

Certain lifestyle habits may be standing in the way of a smaller stomach. Take these tips to heart and results should appear quickly.

Get to Bed Early

> Get enough sleep each night. This will not only provide the body with enough energy to complete workout sessions but will also keep it performing its best all day. Try to get at least 7 hours of restful sleep each night.

Relax

> Keep stress to a minimum. While this is certainly easier said than done, stress is a huge contributor to excess belly fat so consider stress elimination part of a diet.

Take some time each day to refocus and keep life's priorities in order.

Quit Smoking

If someone is a smoker, they should consider the accumulation of belly fat another reason to quit immediately. Many smokers have a large amount of vesicular fat. With healthier lungs, workouts will become more efficient as well.

Stay Hydrated

Drink plenty of water. This will prevent bloating and will help flush away fat causing toxins. It will also keep the body hydrated during exercising and will prevent someone from consuming sugary beverages.

Cut the Caffeine

If several cups of coffee are consumed a day, this can increase the waistline over time, especially if a lot of sugar or flavorings are added. Even if someone drinks black coffee, green tea is a much healthier alternative that can even help him or her lose visceral fat, thanks to compounds called catechins. These compounds can speed up metabolism and help the cells in the stomach release fat.

Break Your Meals Up

When trying to lose belly fat, focus on eating healthier instead of just eating less. Do not skip meals and if hunger strikes in between, it is okay to snack as long as the food is healthy. This will prevent overeating at the end of the day. Experts agree that if possible; break your meals up into 4-6 smaller meals, spread through the day.

Stand Up Straight

Evaluate the body's posture. As the ab muscles strengthen, posture should improve. But begin practicing proper posture now to instantly appear thinner and begin strengthening the spine.

Most importantly, avoid becoming frustrated with while going through this process and transition. If few days of exercise are missed or there is an occasional diet slip up, it does not mean failure has occurred. Keep motivated and if mistakes happen along the way, learn from them and keep moving forward. The ending goal is achievable.

Chapter 5

Exercises

Stop Doing Crunches

Sit-ups or crunches are usually the go to exercise that people do when trying to achieve their goal of getting six pack abs. Most trainers no longer recommend this because of proven negative side effects and the lack of results. Someone can do a million sit-ups and still not see the defined muscle tone that they are after.

The lower the region of the spine is home to important nerves. The spine can also be weakened when excess strain is placed on the area, which is exactly what sit-ups do. The continuous bending required for this exercise damages your back and causes pain and stiffness and can lead to more serious injuries such a herniated disk. Even with a strong back and supporting muscles, sit-ups can still eventually cause injury.

Even if the pain is manageable, the stomach might never have the appearance that someone is after. This is because sit-ups only work the front muscles. While these muscles may improve in appearance, it can leave your stomach with an odd shape since the other ignored muscles will still be undefined. By only focusing on a few of the muscles, the six pack of abs that someone is after will never form. There are several different muscles in the stomach and they all need to be toned together and with the same intensity in order to achieve the goal of a six pack.

Don't Forget About Cardio

Exercises that focus on toning alone though will not provide instant muscle definition. Cardiovascular exercise is important when it comes to burning belly fat too. Begin each workout with some form of cardio. Consider walking, jogging, swimming or aerobics. Any type of high-activity sport will work too, such as basketball or tennis. Keep in mind that one does not need to make a special trip to the gym. Household chores, such as mowing the lawn with a push mower or vigorously vacuuming and dusting can elevate your heart rate and get the body sweating. Whichever activity that is chosen should be done long enough that the heart rate is safely raised for at least 20 minutes. It is also recommended to do the ab workout last during any training session. This is because if they are worked first they will become fatigued and slow down the rest of the workout.

Six Pack Exercises

Side Plank Crunch

The name of this exercise is misleading. It is nothing like the traditional crunches that are not recommended. It will target several of the ab muscles along with strengthening the arms and back. It will also improve balancing skills.

Begin by lying on your left side. Keeping your body straight, push yourself up, balancing your weight between your left foot and left forearm. Place your right hand on your hip and hold your body in a traditional plank pose. Lift your right knee and bring it towards your chest as far as you comfortably can. Do 2 sets of 10 repetitions on each side.

Chair Assisted Plank

This exercise will focus on all of the core muscles and also lift the bottom muscles. Keep the movements slow and uniform in order to benefit the most from this exercise.

Using a sturdy chair, place your hands on each side of it while keeping your arms straight. Take a few steps back and keep your body at an angle, supporting your weight with your arms. Lift your left leg and curl up towards your right arm. Hold for a few seconds and slowly lower your leg back to the ground. Do 10 repetitions on the left side before doing 10 repetitions on the right side. Complete 2 sets.

Leg Lifts

This is a great exercise for beginners since it can be gradually increased in difficulty as progress is made. This exercise reaches the muscles deep in the core that normally are ignored during traditional ab workouts.

Lie on your back with your hands by your side. Slowly lift both legs up towards the ceiling, keeping your body still and controlled. Slowly lower after a few seconds. Repeat until you have done 20 repetitions. Remember that if you are just starting out, it is perfectly okay if you can only do a few. In time you will be able to do the full amount and hold each leg raise longer, increasing the intensity of this exercise.

Bridges

This exercise is almost like a backwards sit-up but without the strain on the back. It also uses different muscles so that the whole core is targeted.

Lie on your back and bend your knees, keeping your feet flat on the floor. Stretch your arms out away from your body. Slowly raise your bottom in the air until your body is holding a right angle at the knees. Hold for a few seconds and slowly lower yourself back to the ground. Complete 3 sets of 15 repetitions each.

Kickbacks

This exercise burns an obscene amount of calories and targets the upper and lower belly regions.

Begin on all fours and keep your back straight but not tight. Bring your belly in and towards your back while you engage your ab muscles. Lift both knees a couple inches off the ground, keeping your balance with your toes. Bring your left knee towards your chin. Immediately kick back with your left leg, keeping it as straight as possible. Be sure to keep your back straight, abs contracted and hips parallel to the floor throughout each movement. Do a set of 8 repetitions on each side for a complete set.

Chapter 6

Recipes

A diet is much more than counting calories and controlling portions. When trying to get rid of stubborn belly fat, it is important to know about the different fats found in food and what they mean for the body.

Saturated fat and trans fat are the ones with a bad reputation and for good reasons. Saturated fat is found mostly in red meat and dairy products. This fat can increase the risk of cardiovascular disease by raising the body's total blood cholesterol levels. Trans fat is sometimes thought of as a man made fat but can be found naturally in certain foods. It is found in dangerous amounts though when food is processed by partial hydrogenation in order to avoid spoiling.

The body does need fat as part of a healthy diet. Some healthier forms of fat include monounsaturated fat, polyunsaturated fat and Omega-3 fatty acids. All of these fats can be consumed naturally. Both monounsaturated and polyunsaturated fats can improve blood cholesterol levels which will lower the risk of developing heart disease. Omega-3 fatty acids are frequently present in fatty fish and is great for the heart. They can also lower blood pressure.

Eggs Italiano

This great breakfast option is a new version of Eggs Benedict that includes fresh vegetables instead of fattening Canadian bacon. Feel free to mix up the vegetables to suit personal taste.

Ingredients:

¼ cup distilled white vinegar

2 teaspoons extra-virgin olive oil

1 shallot, minced

1 clove garlic, minced

2 medium zucchinis, diced

3 plum tomatoes, diced

3 tablespoons sliced fresh basil

1 tablespoon balsamic vinegar

½ teaspoon salt

1 dash ground pepper

8 large eggs

4 whole-wheat English muffins, cut and toasted

2 tablespoons freshly grated Parmesan cheese

Directions:

Fill a tall skillet or Dutch oven with 2 inches of water and bring to a boil. Add the white vinegar.

Heat oil in a separate skillet over medium heat. Add shallot and garlic. Stir while cooking for about 1 minute, or until fragrant. Stir in zucchini and tomatoes and cook until tender, usually about 10 minutes. Remove from heat and stir in 1 tablespoon of the sliced basil, balsamic vinegar, salt and pepper.

Check on the other skillet with the boiling water and lower the heat until there is a gentle simmer. Steam should be coming up from the water and one should see small bubbles emerging from the bottom of the skillet. One by one, crack each egg into a small bowl and transfer gently into the water. Avoid breaking any yolks. Cook for 4-8 minutes, depending on preferred taste. Carefully remove each egg with a slotted spoon and place on a paper towel to drain.

To prepare for serving, top each toasted muffin half with vegetables, an egg, Parmesan cheese and the remaining basil.

Creamy Fettuccine with Brussels Sprouts and Mushrooms

Even when on a diet, one can still enjoy delicious pasta with a creamy sauce. Being able to healthily indulge will keep someone from sabotaging their diet.

Ingredients:

12 ounces whole-wheat fettuccine

1 tablespoon extra-virgin olive oil

4 cups sliced mushrooms (shitake or cremini are suggested but can be any variety)

4 cups thinly sliced Brussels sprouts

1 tablespoon minced garlic

½ cup dry sherry

2 cups low-fat milk

2 tablespoons all-purpose flour

½ teaspoon salt

½ teaspoon freshly ground pepper

1 cup shredded Asiago cheese

Directions:

Cook pasta according to cooking directions. Drain and return to pot and set aside.

In a large skillet, heat oil over medium heat. Cook Brussels sprouts and mushrooms, stirring often, until tender, usually 8-10 minutes. Add garlic and cook for 1 minute. Add sherry and scrape pan to loosen any brown bits. Bring liquid to a boil and continuously stir until the liquid has almost all evaporated.

Whisk milk and flour in a separate bowl. Add salt and pepper and slowly incorporate into the skillet. Cook until the sauce begins to bubble. It should thicken within 2 minutes. Mix in Asiago and cook until melted. Transfer the sauce to the pasta and mix.

Steak and Pepper Tacos

This is a light yet filling meal. Feel free to double the recipe so that everyone in the family can have leftovers for lunch the next day.

Ingredients:

1 pound flank steak

1 lime, juiced

1 teaspoon kosher salt

2 crushed garlic cloves

½ teaspoon chili powder

3 teaspoons vegetable oil

½ red onion, sliced

3 bell peppers of preferred color, sliced into thin strips

½ cup corn kernels

8 small corn tortillas

1 avocado, sliced

¼ cup Monterrey Jack cheese

2 tablespoons chopped fresh cilantro

1-2 jalapenos, sliced

Reduced fat sour cream, if desired

Directions:

Combine lime juice, salt, garlic and chili powder. Marinate the steak in the mixture.

Heat 2 teaspoons of vegetable oil in a large skillet. Add onion and bell peppers and cook until tender. Add the corn and cook an additional 2 minutes. Remove the vegetables from the skillet and keep warm. Add the last teaspoon of vegetable oil and add the marinated steak. Cook for about 8 minutes or longer if a more well steak is desired. Remove from the skillet and allow to rest for several minutes.

Slice the steak and add to vegetables. Assemble tacos with desired toppings.

Spinach-Mushroom Pizza

This is a great and healthy alternative to traditional pizza that will satisfy the taste buds.

Ingredients:

1 12 ounce whole wheat pizza crust

¼ cup pizza sauce

½ cup frozen spinach, thawed and drained

¼ red onion, thinly sliced

1 cup shredded part-skim mozzarella cheese

6 cremini mushrooms, sliced

¼ cup part-skim ricotta cheese

2 tablespoons grated Parmesan

1 tablespoon extra-virgin olive oil

2 teaspoons balsamic vinegar

Directions:

Preheat the over to 450 degrees Fahrenheit. Lay the pizza crust out. Pour and spread the pizza sauce on the crust. Top with the spinach and onion. Continue with placing the mushrooms and mozzarella. Top with the ricotta cheese and sprinkle with the Parmesan. Drizzle the olive oil over the whole pizza.

Place the pizza on the baking sheet that has been warming in the oven. Bake for 10 minutes, or until the cheese has melted and the crust has puffed up and taken on color. Turn on the oven's broiler and broil the pizza for another couple of minutes, or until cheese is just starting to brown. Allow the pizza to cool and sprinkle with the balsamic vinegar. Slice and serve.

Cumin Salmon with Yogurt-Cucumber Sauce

A light yet filling meal that will satisfy seafood cravings. It is also quick to make so it works great as a dinner for when time is limited.

Ingredients:

2 teaspoons extra-virgin olive oil

½ teaspoon ground cumin

½ teaspoon sugar

½ teaspoon black pepper

½ teaspoon salt

4 salmon fillets, approximately 4 ounces each

½ cup nonfat Greek yogurt

1 large pickling cucumber, peeled, seeded and diced

1 scallion, trimmed and chopped

3 tablespoons minced fresh parsley

1 teaspoon fresh lemon juice

8 ounces whole wheat orzo, cooked according to package directions

Directions:

Combine the olive oil, cumin, sugar, black pepper and salt in a small bowl. Place the salmon on a baking sheet lined with aluminum foil and brush each fillet with the oil mixture. Preheat the oven's broiler. In another bow, combine the yogurt, cucumber, scallion, parsley, and lemon juice. Broil the salmon for 7-10 minutes or until the thickest areas are cooked thoroughly. Serve the fillets over the prepared orzo and top with the yogurt sauce.

Feel free to modify these recipes slightly to cater to personal taste preferences using the list of belly fat blasting foods as a guide to substitutes. Remember that a diet is more easily followed with a little wiggle room but keep the bad foods and fats in moderation. Once one learns how to eat healthier instead of only cutting down on portion sizes, they will be able to come up with their own recipes and also find ways to modify their favorite dishes.

Conclusion

Belly fat can be a frustrating and esteem-crushing problem and has only become more common over the years. Easily accessible unhealthy food and a lifestyle that promotes less physical work is a combination that sets up for larger midsections.

However, with proper nutrition and effective exercises, you can now make belly fat a thing of the past and never have to worry about it coming back. You can live each day more confident and enjoy the health benefits that come with having a trim and fit stomach.

Start incorporating the lessons and advice that you have learned from this book into your life today. Try one of the recipes for dinner or start learning some of the exercises when you get home instead of sitting on the couch right away. By doing a little more each day and slowly incorporating new and healthier habits into your daily life, you will soon be seeing results that will be motivation enough to continue on your journey. Once people notice your weight loss and muscle definition, they will want to know all of your secrets.

Note from the Publisher:

We hope you've found plenty of useful information within these pages! Green Ribbon Engagements is dedicated to creating engaging content that is meant to help people. To view more of our books, please visit our website.

http://www.greenribbonengagements.com/epublishing.html

We'd love to know what you thought! Leave us a review if you found this quick guide helpful!